Copyrighted Material

This book or parts thereof may not be reproduced in any form whatsoever, store or transmitted by any means-electronic, photocopy, mechanical, recording or otherwise, without prior permission of the publisher.

Copyright @2018 by Jane Lordson

All right reserved

Diabetes: Simple Home Remedies

Table of Content

Diabetes in perspective	4
Different types of Diabetes	6
What is type I Diabetes?	6
What is type II Diabetes?	9
Other types of Diabetes	11
Causes of Diabetes	14
Common symptoms of Diabetes	18
Chronic complications of Diabetes	19

Diabetes: Simple Home Remedies

Herbal and natural Diabetes Therapies	22
Simple home remedies for Diabetes	23
Things to avoid	59
Diets remedies for Diabetes	60

Diabetes: Simple Home Remedies

Diabetes in perspective:

Diabetes is a disease that is synonymous with high blood sugar (glucose) levels that result from deficiency in insulin secretion. In the olden days, diabetes was first identified as a "sweet urine" disease and excessive muscle loss. High levels of blood glucose lead to spillage of glucose into the urine, thus the name sweet urine.

Blood glucose levels are normally regulated by insulin, a hormone secreted by the pancreas. The major function of insulin is to lowers the blood glucose level. When the blood glucose rises (e.g. after exercise), insulin is secreted from the pancreas to stabilize the glucose level by inducing the flow of glucose into the body system. It must be noted that low secretion of, or lack of response to insulin causes hyperglycemia in patients with diabetes. Diabetes is a chronic medical

Diabetes: Simple Home Remedies

condition in human, though it can be controlled but it can also last a lifetime.

United States diabetes figures

- In recent years, diabetes has been identified as the 7th leading cause of death in the United States as listed on death certificates.

- In the United States, approximately 29.1 million people (9.3% of the population) have diabetes, while another 86 million people have pre-diabetes and they are not aware of it.

- Also, about 8.1 million people have diabetes and don't even know it.

- In the long run, diabetes can result to serious conditions like; blindness, kidney failure, and nerve damage.

- Diabetes is also an important factor in increasing the narrowing and hardening of the arteries resulting into strokes, blood vessel

Diabetes: Simple Home Remedies

and coronary heart disease. This is refers to as macro vascular disease.

- Medical expenses for people with diabetes are over two times higher than those for people who do not have diabetes. Remember, these numbers reflect only the population in the United States.

Different types of Diabetes

Basically, we have two major types of diabetes and they are often refers to as type 1 and type 2. Type 1 diabetes can also be refers to as insulin dependent diabetes, or as juvenile-onset diabetes. Type 1 diabetes is associated with a situation where the pancreas goes through an autoimmune attack by the body itself, and is rendered incapable of insulin secretion. Abnormal antibodies have been discovered in many patients with type 1 diabetes. Antibodies serve as proteins in the blood and form an integral part of the body's immune system. Type 1 diabetes patients always rely on insulin treatment for survival.

What is type 1 diabetes

In disease like type 1 diabetes, the immune system produce antibodies that are directed at foreign body's agents causing damage to the body tissues of the patients. In type 1 diabetes patients, the cells which are responsible for insulin production (beta cells of the pancreas), are attacked by the misdirected immune system. The tendency of developing abnormal antibodies in type 1 diabetes has been generally associated to genetic inheritance.

Exposure to viral infections and environmental toxins can as well cause abnormal antibody responses that may result into damage to the pancreas cells where insulin is produce. Some of the antibodies present in type 1 diabetes include;

- Anti-insulin antibodies
- Anti-glutamic decarboxylase
- Antibodies
- Anti-islet cell antibodies.

These antibodies are present in the majority of patients, and can assist in determining individuals at risk for developing type 1 diabetes.

Type 1 diabetes usually occurs among young individuals, mostly before 30 years of age. However, this form of diabetes does occur among the older people, but on a rare occasion. This type of condition in adult subgroup is known as latent autoimmune diabetes in adults, which is a progressive form of type 1 diabetes. Among all the people with diabetes, just only 10 percent have type 1 diabetes, the rest 90 percent have type 2 diabetes.

What is type 2 diabetes?

Type 2 diabetes can also be refers to as non-insulin dependent diabetes. In type 2 diabetes, insulin can still be produced by patient, but on a low level which is inadequate for the body's needs. Though In some instances, the pancreas secretes more than normal quantities of insulin required by the body. A common trait of type 2 diabetes is a lack of sensitivity to insulin by the body cells.

In addition, the release of insulin by the pancreas may also be low and defective compare to the body's need. There is an established fact of steady decline in beta cell secretion of insulin in type 2 diabetes that worsens glucose control.

While it is a fact that type 2 diabetes occurs mostly in adult individuals and this incidence increases with age. It is interesting to note that increase numbers of patients with type 2 diabetes are barely in their teen. Majority of these cases are a direct result of lack of exercise and poor eating habits. Other risk factor that encourages the developing this form of diabetes is obesity and this is common among children as well as adults. It is estimated that the probability of developing diabetes multiply by 20% for every increase in body weight.

In relation to age, research shows that there is an increase in incidence of diabetes at every decade after 40 years of age regardless of body weight. Diabetes occurrence tendency is high as much as 26% in persons of 65 years of age and above. Type 2 diabetes is also common among certain ethnic groups, and also develops frequently in women with a prior history of gestational diabetes.

Other types of diabetes

Gestational diabetes:

This diabetes occurs temporarily during pregnancy, and study has shown that it occurs in 2% to 10% of all pregnancies. Little change in hormones during pregnancy can lead to increase in blood sugar level of individuals. Increase in blood sugar during pregnancy is refers to as gestational diabetes. Gestational diabetes normally disappears once the baby is born. However, there is a high probability of 35% to 60% of women with gestational diabetes to later develop type II diabetes in the next one to two decades, majorly those that are overweight during pregnancy and after delivery and those that require insulin during pregnancy are susceptible to this condition.

Secondary diabetes:

Another type of diabetes is secondary diabetes which refers to increase in blood sugar levels as a result of other medical condition. This form of diabetes develops when the pancreatic tissues are destroyed by disease. The pancreas majorly produces insulin for body needs.

Diabetes: Simple Home Remedies

Diabetes: Facts

- Diabetes is a serious condition associated with abnormal high levels of sugar in the blood system. Pancreas produces insulin which lowers blood sugar (glucose).
- Diabetes is caused by the insufficient production or the absence of insulin, or an inability of the body to properly use the available insulin.

  Generally, diabetes is of two types, namely;

  -Type 1 diabetes or insulin dependent (common in teens and children)

  -Type 2 diabetes or non-insulin dependent (common in adults)

Causes diabetes

The major causes of diabetes are;

-Insufficient insulin production or secretion, relative to the body's needs.

- Secretion or production of defective insulin which is not usually common.

-The inability of the body cells to use insulin optimally, may also leads to diabetes.

- The latter condition affects mostly the fat tissues and cells, and results in a condition known as insulin resistance. This is the major problem in type 2 diabetes.

Diabetes: Simple Home Remedies

- The main disorder in type 1 diabetes is lack of insulin which is part of the destructive process affecting the insulin-secretion beta cell in the pancreas.

Type 2 diabetes also has a steady reduction of beta cells that contribute to the process of increased blood sugars. Importantly, the body can to some extent boosts the production of insulin and overcome the level of resistance in a situation someone is resistant to insulin. Over time, if insulin secretion reduces and cannot be released vigorously as expected, diabetes develops.

Glucose:

Glucose in a clear term is a sugar found in food. Glucose is an important nutrient that gives energy for proper functioning of the body system. The glucose in food is absorbed by the intestinal cells into the bloodstream after the food must have been digested, and it is transport by the bloodstream to all the necessary cells in the body where it is properly used. However, glucose needs insulin to enter the cells, without insulin the cells are deprived of glucose energy. In some types of diabetes, the inability of the cell to used up the glucose result into those glucose being pass out as excreted urine.

INSULIN:

Insulin is a hormone produced by the pancreas. (The pancreas is an organ in the abdomen right behind the stomach). Insulin apart from assisting the glucose in entering the cell is also vital in controlling the glucose in the blood. In a diabetics patients, insulin is either relatively insufficient for the body's needs, absent or not properly used by the body. All these cause increase levels of blood glucose.

Risk factors for diabetes

Diabetes: Simple Home Remedies

Risk factors for type 1 diabetes are not well comprehended as those for type 2 diabetes. Family health history is a major known risk factor for type 1 diabetes. Other risk factors for diabetes may include having certain diseases or infections of the pancreas.

Risk factors for Type 2 diabetes and pre-diabetes are numerous. Among those risks factor that can raise the risk of developing type II diabetes are:

- Family history
- Increasing age
- Being obese or overweight
- Gestational diabetes during a pregnancy
- High blood pressure
- Sedentary lifestyle
- Ethnic background

Diabetes: Simple Home Remedies

- Insulin resistance

- Impaired glucose tolerance

- Polycystic ovary syndrome

Common symptoms of diabetes

- Fatigue

- Numbness in the feet or toes

- hunger

- blurred vision

- increase urine output

- slow healing wounds, sores or cuts

- fatigue

- nausea

- Yeast infections

Diabetes: Simple Home Remedies

- Dehydration
- weight loss or gain
- skin problems
- Frequent infections
- Dry mouth

Chronic complications of diabetes

Eye Complications:

Eye complication of diabetes is refers to as diabetic retinopathy and it is mostly happen in patients with diabetes history for at least five years. Leakage of protein, formation of small aneurysms in the eye can be caused by disease in the blood vessels of the eye. Bleeding caused by this disease can lead to impaired vision, cataracts and glaucoma.

Diabetes: Simple Home Remedies

Kidney damage:

The beginning of kidney disease and its progression is extremely different. Leakage of protein in the urine can be caused by diseased small blood vessels in the kidney which Later make the kidneys to lose its ability to cleanse and filter blood. This may result into the need for dialysis as result of accumulation of toxic waste products in the blood.

Nerve damage:

Diabetic neuropathy is a name associated with nerve damage from diabetic and it occurs as a result of disease of small blood vessels. There is limited blood flow to the nerves thereby leaving the nerves shortage of blood flow thus cause severe damage in the process. Loss of sensation in the feet is a major symptom of diabetic nerve damage. Other symptoms includes; feet aching, feet numbness and burning.

Diabetes: Simple Home Remedies

Diabetic nerve damage can also result into erectile dysfunction and lead to impotence.

Exercise:

Overweight is one of the major reasons for type II diabetes. Exercise of any kind can helps in improving blood sugar level and keeping the right weight. Daily walking and jogging can also help in reducing the blood sugar level.

Herbal and Natural Diabetes Therapies

Most common herbs and spices contain blood sugar lowering properties that are useful for managing and treating type II diabetes.

Diabetes: Simple Home Remedies

A lot of research has been conducted on the potency of those herbs and spices in improving blood glucose level as well as diabetes management. The outcome shows a fantastic and perfect result.

The available herbal therapies:

Some herbs and spices contain antioxidant properties that have great potential in treating and managing diabetes. Some of these herbs include;

- Okra
- Fenugreek
- Aloe Vera
- Cinnamon
- Bilberry extract
- Bitter melon
- Cherries

Diabetes: Simple Home Remedies

- Ginger
- Avocado
- Bitter gourd
- Holy basil
- Etc

Simple Home Remedies for Diabetes

1. Guava

Guava trees are grown widely in many countries and its leaves and fruits are considered as highly medicinal because of its numerous health benefits. Guava leaves extract has been found to be effective remedy for diabetes mellitus. Flavonoid presence in guava increases its ability to reduce blood sugar. The guava fruits and leaves have

Diabetes: Simple Home Remedies

more than ten substances that fight against diabetes. Some active properties in guava includes; fructose, pectin fiber, ursolic acid, zinc, magnesium, niacin and manganese.

Eating fresh guava fruits regularly can help in treating diabetes. It is advisable for diabetes patients to peel off the skin of guava fruits before consumption. Guava tea can also help in treating diabetes and this can be made with guava leaves. The procedure below can be follow in making the guava tea.

- Get guava leaves in a clean tray.
- Pour 1 to 2 cups of water on the leaves.
- Boil it for a couple of minutes until the water is half dried.
- Strain the water after turning off the heat.
- Allow the tea to cool down to the room temperature.
- Drink two to three glass cups daily.

Diabetes: Simple Home Remedies

2. Apples

The risk of developing diabetes can be reduced by regular consumption of apples. Research has shown great improvement in diabetes patients after eating apple regularly over a period of time. Apple fruits are abundantly rich in soluble fiber, antioxidants and vitamin C. The presence of pectin in apples helps in removing toxin waste from the body system and stabilizing the insulin level. Daily consumption of medium size apple is encouraged for slowing down the development of diabetes.

3. Cherries

Cherries are unique fruit loaded with beta-carotene, vitamin C, antioxidants, iron, potassium, fiber, folate and magnesium. The presence of anthocyanins in cherries can increase production by up to fifty percent and this help in lowering blood pressure as well

Diabetes: Simple Home Remedies

as improving diabetes condition. Aside diabetes control, cherries consumption can combat heart disease, cancer and other health problems associated with a cancer's patient.

Direction for cherries consumption:

Cherries can be consumed fresh, dried, frozen or canned. It can also be made into juice. Half glass juice cup should be consumed daily.

4. Grapefruit

Grapefruit has been identified and recommended as diabetes super food by the American Diabetes Association. The fruit is rich in soluble fiber, vitamin C and naringenin (flavonoid) which makes the body sensitive to insulin and helps in keeping the right weight.

Diabetes: Simple Home Remedies

To get the best out of grapefruit, the fruit should be process into juice and one glass cup should be consumed daily.

5. Avocado

Avocado contains high amount of mono-unsaturated fat and fiber which is highly beneficial in managing body blood sugar, improving the heart health and preventing heart disease. For optimum result, diabetes patients are encouraged to consume a medium avocado daily. Avocado can also be added to salads and sandwiches.

6. Strawberries

Strawberries contain fiber, vitamins and strong antioxidants that help in lowering bad cholesterol and promoting the good cholesterol thereby reducing the severity of diabetes. Strawberries should be taken as snacks by diabetes patients or it can be added to cereals and salads.

7. Oranges

Oranges are rich in fiber, vitamin C and essential mineral like thiamin that is good in controlling diabetes. The glycemic presence in orange regulates the release of glucose into the blood stream. In addition, weight gain is being control by regular consumption of oranges thereby eliminating overweight and obesity as a risk factor of developing diabetes. Consumption of one to two oranges per day is strongly recommended. It is more beneficial to consume orange in their natural form than extracting juice from them. You tend to get more fiber from consuming oranges in their natural form than drinking orange juice.

Diabetes: Simple Home Remedies

8. Pears

Pears are loaded with vitamin A, B1, B2, C and E. Pears consumption can boost the immune system, control blood sugar levels, improve digestive health and improve the immune system. Type 2 diabetes patient are encourage to eat pears regularly because of its insulin sensitivity. Eating of one medium sized of pears daily is good in reliving diabetes.

9. Kiwi

Kiwi is a healthy fruit and it is rich in beta-carotene, vitamin A, E, flavonoids and potassium that help in improving the immune system. The low carbohydrate content in kiwi is good sources of fiber that help in regulating blood sugar level and lower cholesterol. One kiwi a day is healthy for the body.

Diabetes: Simple Home Remedies

10. Olive Oil

Olive oil is good in reducing blood sugar level thus aid in diabetes control. It can be use as alternative to cooking oil or as salad dressings ingredients. As a result of its high calories, there should be limit in the daily amount of olive oil use.

11. Pear Cactus Juice

Cactus juice is one the cheaper way of getting fiber and serves as remedies for diabetes. The fiber contain in cactus juice have the ability of slowing down the process of sugar absorption in the body and put the glucose level under check. Pear cactus juice is rich in iron, vitamin A, C, E, calcium, carotenoids as well as contains both the anti-inflammatory and anti-viral properties.

Diabetes: Simple Home Remedies

Prickly pear cactus juice methods and procedure

Ingredients needed:

- 2 cup of water.
- 1 peeled and chooped cucumber.
- 2 juice lime.
- ½ peeled and chopped cucumber..

The procedure:

- Blend all the ingredients with blender.
- Sieve to get the juice.
- Drink daily for a week.

Diabetes: Simple Home Remedies

12. Bilberry

Bilberry plant has been around for sometimes, and its leaves have been found to be effective in reducing blood sugar level. The plant contains an anthocyanidin which is potent in treating diabetes and ulcers. Among the numerous antioxidants properties in bilberry are; phenolic compounds, hydroxycinnamic acids, vitamin A, vitamin C, catechins and proanthocyanidins. The role of antioxidants is to guide the body cell from damages associated with free radicals.

Dried or fresh bilberry can be process into syrup or tea and take regularly. To make a bilberry tea, the following procedures are involved.

- Boil water in a kettle.

Diabetes: Simple Home Remedies

- Get a dried bilberry.

- Put a tablespoon (dried bilberry) in a mug.

- Pour hot water over it.

- Cover it for ten minutes.

- Drink two to three glass cup daily.

Other health benefits of bilberry:

- Improve blood circulation

- Strengthens blood vessels

- Treats diarrhea

- Help in treating retinopathy.

- Prevent cell damage

Diabetes: Simple Home Remedies

13. Green Tea

Among the benefits of green are;

-Lowering the risk of developing certain form of cancer.

-Slowing down the aging process.

-Boosting the immune system.

-Protecting the body from bacteria.

-Improving the cardiovascular health.

Aside these, the green tea have also been found to help in increasing the body's sensitiveness to insulin thereby improving the metabolism function. Green tea has also been found to contain polyphenols which has the ability of reducing cholesterol, preventing blood cloth and lowering blood pressure. The polyphenols in green tea is also good in maintaining the body glucose level, thus helps in treating and preventing diabetes. Drinking five cups of green tea daily is recommended in reducing the risk of type II diabetes.

14. Drumstick Leaves

Drumstick leaves is highly acknowledge for its medicinal values, and it has been in use for ages to treat many ailments (diabetes inclusive). The anti-inflammation properties of drumstick leaves are good in detoxifying the body system, increasing body metabolism and controlling blood sugar level.

To use drumstick leaves for diabetes, you can do this:

- Get a mix grinder ready.
- Get some fresh drumstick leaves.
- Put the drumsticks in the mixer grinder and add a little water.

Diabetes: Simple Home Remedies

- Gently blend together.

- Get the juice from the drumsticks leaves by straining the pulp.

- Drink half one cup of the juice daily for three weeks.

You should be able to see a significant improvement in blood sugar level within this period.

15. Fenugreek

Fenugreek assists in promoting pancreas cells thereby boosting insulin production. To get the best out of fenugreek, use any of this method:

Method 1:

- 8 tablespoons of fenugreek seeds
- 2 cups of water

Diabetes: Simple Home Remedies

The process:

- Put Fenugreek seeds in a bowl.
- Soak in water overnight.
- Get the seeds out in the morning and crush.
- Strain and get the water.
- Drink the water twice a day for a period of 8 weeks.

Method: 2:

- Get some quantity of water.
- 4 tablespoons of fenugreek seeds.

The process:

- Put Fenugreek seeds in a bowl.
- Soak in water overnight.

Diabetes: Simple Home Remedies

- Consume the soaked fenugreek seeds by chewing the next morning and drink the water along with the seeds.
- To get maximum result, take this solution on an empty stomach.
- Repeat this process for 8 weeks.

Method 3:

- Get 2 glass of milk or warm water.
- 4 tablespoons of fenugreek seeds powder

The process:

- Add fenugreek seeds powder in milk or warm water.
- Stir the mixture and drink the solution to get relief from the diabetes.
- This process should be repeated daily for 8 weeks for effective result.

Diabetes: Simple Home Remedies

Method 4:

- 1½ tablespoons of turmeric powder.
- 3 tablespoons of fenugreeks seeds.
- White pepper.
- 1 ½ glass of milk.

The process:

- Get fenugreek seeds into a bowl.
- Add little turmeric powder and white pepper.
- Mix thoroughly and grind into powder.
- Add a teaspoon of the powder to the milk.
- Mix thoroughly and drink thrice daily.

Diabetes: Simple Home Remedies

16. Bitter Gourd

Bitter gourd is a class of vegetable that is healthy and serve as remedy for diabetes especially the type 2 diabetes. Apart from diabetes, bitter gourd is also good for fighting variety of disease and infection. Below are various ways to get the best out of bitter gourd:

Method 1:

The needed materials:

- Peeler
- Water
- Bitter gourd – 6
- Sieve

Diabetes: Simple Home Remedies

The process:

- Peel the bitter gourds.
- Cut the gourds into pieces and remove the seeds.
- Create paste from the deseeded peeled bitter gourd by crushing.
- Sieve the solution by squeezing and extract the juice
- Drink the juice on an empty stomach every morning for two weeks.

Method 2:

Materials needed:

- Clarified butter.
- Bitter gourd
- Pan

The process:

Diabetes: Simple Home Remedies

- Cut the bitter gourd into pieces.
- Add clarified butter into a pan and pour the bitter gourd in the pan.
- Cook for some minutes.
- Eat this once a day for three months.

Method 3:

- One cup of water
- Some pieces of dried bitter melon
- Pan

The Process:

- Boil water in a pot for few minutes and add some dried bitter melon.
- Mix properly and sieve to get the tea

Diabetes: Simple Home Remedies

- Drink the tea every morning for six to eight weeks.

17. Neem Leaves

The neem contains anti-bacterial, antifungal and anti-hyperglycemic that is good in boosting insulin production, lowering blood glucose level and diabetes treatment.

Method 1:

- Get some fresh neem leaves.
- Extract juice from the leave by crushing and strain the water.
- Take 1 teaspoon of the juice every morning for 6-8 weeks on an empty stomach.

  Method 2:

- 10-12 leaves of Neem leaves

Diabetes: Simple Home Remedies

The Process:

- Get some tender neem leaves and wash properly.
- Chew this every morning.
- Repeat the process every morning till you notice some level of improvement.

Method 3:

- 2 to 4 teaspoon of dried neem leaves powder
- 2 glass of water

The Process:

- Add the powder in some water.
- Stir thoroughly to get a well blended solution.
- Drink the solution every morning till you get a noticeable improvement.

Diabetes: Simple Home Remedies

18. Holy Basil

Holy basil has numerous healthy properties like; anti-viral, anti-stress, anti-fungal, anti-bacterial, antioxidants, anti-ulcer, immune stimulant and anti-diabetes. To get optimum benefit of holy basil, any of the following method can be use:

Method 1:

- Water
- 3-6 leaves of Fresh basil leaves

The Process:

- Wash the basil leaves properly.
- Chew them on an empty stomach in the morning.
- Repeat the process for 4-8 weeks.

Method 2:

Diabetes: Simple Home Remedies

- Vegetable juice or water.
- Basil leaves.

The process:

- Extract juice from basil leaves by crushing.
- Add water or vegetable juice to the basil juice.
- Stir properly and drink on an empty stomach every morning.
- Repeat the process for 6-8 weeks.

Method 3:

- Beat leaves-4
- Basil leaves – 4
- Neem leaves – 4

The process:

- Get a neem leaves, basil and beat leaves.

- Crush together to get a paste
- Take the paste on an empty stomach every morning for 6-8 weeks.

19. Flaxseeds

Flaxseeds usage is also one of the best remedies for diabetes treatment and management. Flaxseed is rich in fiber, protein and lignans, which act as anti-oxidants. Also, flaxseeds can help in stabilizing blood sugar level. To get the best out of flaxseed, any of the methods below can be use.

Method 1:

- Get one glass cup of milk or water
- 1 tablespoon of flaxseed powder.

The process:

Diabetes: Simple Home Remedies

- Add flaxseed powder in warm water.

- Stir properly and drink daily (morning) for 6-8 weeks

- Take warm milk or water and then add flaxseed powder in this.

Method 2:

- Get 1 tablespoon of flaxseed powder

The process:

- Add the flaxseed powder into the breakfast cereal and have it as breakfast.

- Regular intake of this meal can help you control diabetes.

20. Papaya Leaf

Papaya leaf is a good home remedy for diabetes mellitus. The leaf is useful in increasing the insulin production and sensitivity. Papaya leaf

Diabetes: Simple Home Remedies

can be use in treating diabetes in many ways but the simplest one is discussed below.

- Papaya leaves – 5
- cups of water -4
- Cooking pot

The process:

- Pour some water in a cooking pot and place it on the heat.
- Add the papaya leaves to the water.
- Allow the water to boil for some minutes (10-15 minutes).
- Take a pan and next pour water in this and place it on the heat or stove.
- Allow the solution to cool down then filter the water.
- Drink daily for 2-4 weeks.

Diabetes: Simple Home Remedies

21. Lady's Finger

Lady's finger is also known as okra. It contains great amount of useful vitamin like B6, C,A,K, magnesium, zinc, potassium, fiber and polyphenolic molecules that reduces the blood glucose level as well as fighting diabetes in the body. Below is the okra guide for diabetes treatment.

- Get 3-6 okra or lady's finger
- 1 glass of Water

The process:

- Rinse the okra in a clean water
- Gently cut the head and tail of the okra to get two pieces from each lady-s finger (slit it vertically from the middle).
- Soak these pieces in covered water overnight.

Diabetes: Simple Home Remedies

- Drink the water first thing in the morning before any food.

- Lady's finger can be equally incorporated in a daily diet

- Repeat the process for 4-8 weeks to get an optimum result.

22. Mango Leaves

Mango laves are simple home remedy for diabetes that has been in existence for ages. It can be use through any of the methods highlighted below:

Method 1:

- One glass of water

- 8-12 Mango leaves

- Sieve or strain.

The process:

- Clean the mango leaves by rinsing.

Diabetes: Simple Home Remedies

- Place the leaves in a cooking pot and cover with water
- Soak it over night and filter the water in the morning.
- Drink on an empty stomach in the morning.
- Have breakfast one hour after drinking.
- Repeat this process 4-6 weeks.

Method 2:

- Get dried Mango leaves
- Get a clean Container

The process:

- Blend or grind the mango leaves into powder form and keep in a container.
- Use the powder as a tea (1/2 teaspoon) before lunch.
- Repeat the process 4- weeks.

Diabetes: Simple Home Remedies

23. Aloe Vera

Never look past Aloe Vera when next you are looking for the best home remedy for diabetes. Aloe Vera can be use to manage and cure diabetes as follows:

Method 1:

- ½ tablespoon of bay leaves powder.
- ½ tablespoon of Aloe Vera gel.
- ½ tablespoon of turmeric powder.

The process:

- Mix all the ingredients together in a bowl in equal quantities.
- Take the mixture before lunch
- Repeat the process for 6-8 weeks.

Method 2:

Diabetes: Simple Home Remedies

The process:

- Aloe Vera juice- 1 tablespoon
- Buttermilk - I glass

The process:

- Add Aloe Vera gel in the buttermilk.
- Mix together and stir thoroughly and drink every morning.

24. Curry Leaves

Curry leaves possess high amount of mineral like copper, iron and zinc that help in regulating glucose level in the blood. Curry leaves can be use in the following ways to manage diabetes.

Method 1:

- Fresh leaves of curry (6-10 pieces)

Diabetes: Simple Home Remedies

The process:

- Wash the curry leaves properly.
- Chew gently and repeat the process once daily for 6 weeks.

Method 2:

- Curry leaves

The process:

- Wash the curry leaves and add in your cooking.
- They can be added to salad and sauces.

Diabetes: Simple Home Remedies

25. Cinnamon

Cinnamon has also been found to be effective in treating diabetes. Cinnamon powder is good in stimulating insulin activity and lowering of blood sugar.

To use cinnamon:

- Add one tablespoon of cinnamon powder into one cup of hot water.
- Allow it to cool before dinking.
- Cinnamon powder can also be sprinkle on salad or mix with soup.
- Cinnamon powder can also be added to coffee, milk or tea.

Diabetes: Simple Home Remedies

26- Garlic

Garlic contains strong antioxidant properties and micro-circulatory effects. Garlic has shown great effect in reducing blood glucose and boost insulin secretion.

Other benefits of garlic include:

- Good in treating constipation
- Aid digestive health
- Good for dental health
- Heal post surgery scars

27- Bitter Melon

Bitter melon is a unique vegetable that have a superb ability to reduce blood glucose level as well as treating various ailments. Bitter melon is rich in vitamins, minerals and some antioxidants property. Bitter melon contains three active properties: polypeptide-p, vicine and charantin.

Diabetes: Simple Home Remedies

These properties are useful in lowering blood glucose level and treating type 2 diabetes. Bitter melon is also good in treating other ailments like;

- Burns
- Colic
- Skin conditions
- Cough
- Fever
- Painful menstruation

Home remedies for diabetes treatment

Things to avoid:

1. GMO products - GMO foods and products have the tendency of

increasing diabetes as well as causing kidney and liver diseases. It is advisable to consume food labeled as GMO-free.

2. Refined sugar –Sugar is generally bad for diabetes patients because of the direct role it play in blood sugar level's position. So, it is advisable to avoid refined sugar by all means.

3. Alcohol – Apart from damaging the liver, alcohol consumption also affects the pancreas and the insulin production. Thus, alcoholic consumption should be greatly reduced if not totally avoided.

4. Whole grains –Grains that contains gluten should be avoided. Gluten is link with diabetes and its consumption can result into inflammation and trigger other health complications.

Diabetes: Simple Home Remedies

5. Cow milk – It is advisable for diabetes patients to avoid cow milk as it can trigger the immune system and lead to inflammation. Goat and sheep milk should be consumed instead as its helps to maintain blood sugar level.

Diet Remedies for Diabetes

For the expected results, you need to:

- Cut down on high carbohydrate foods like yam, sweet potatoes and oily food.
- Do away with refined flour; rather use whole wheat pasta instead of using whole grains.

Diabetes: Simple Home Remedies

- Make juices out of carrot, pomegranate and pumpkin drink 1 glass every morning.

- Use more of low dairy products like yogurt, cheese and skimmed milk.

- Incorporate spinach, bitter gourd, onion, raw banana and garlic in diet.

- Do away with sweet fruits like grapes and pineapples.

- Reduce salt intake to the barest minimum.

- Mix 1 teaspoon of garlic juice and the same amount of ginger juice with honey and take this daily on an empty stomach.

Lastly, to keep diabetes at bay ensures you keep a healthy diet, engage in regular exercise, medication, and good mood.

Diabetes: Simple Home Remedies